Illustrated Animal Poetry

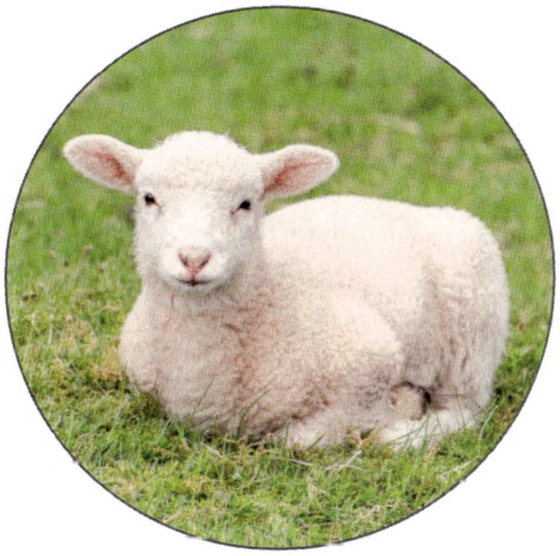

This book of verses from long-ago classic poems belongs to:

____

Hurt no living thing

Hurt no living thing:
Ladybird, nor butterfly,
Nor moth with dusty wing,
Nor cricket chirping cheerily,
Nor grasshopper so light of leap,
Nor dancing gnat, nor beetle fat,
Nor harmless worms that creep.

Christina Rossetti

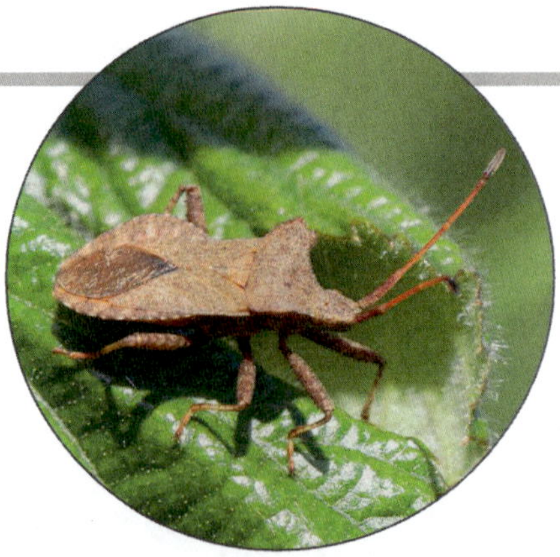

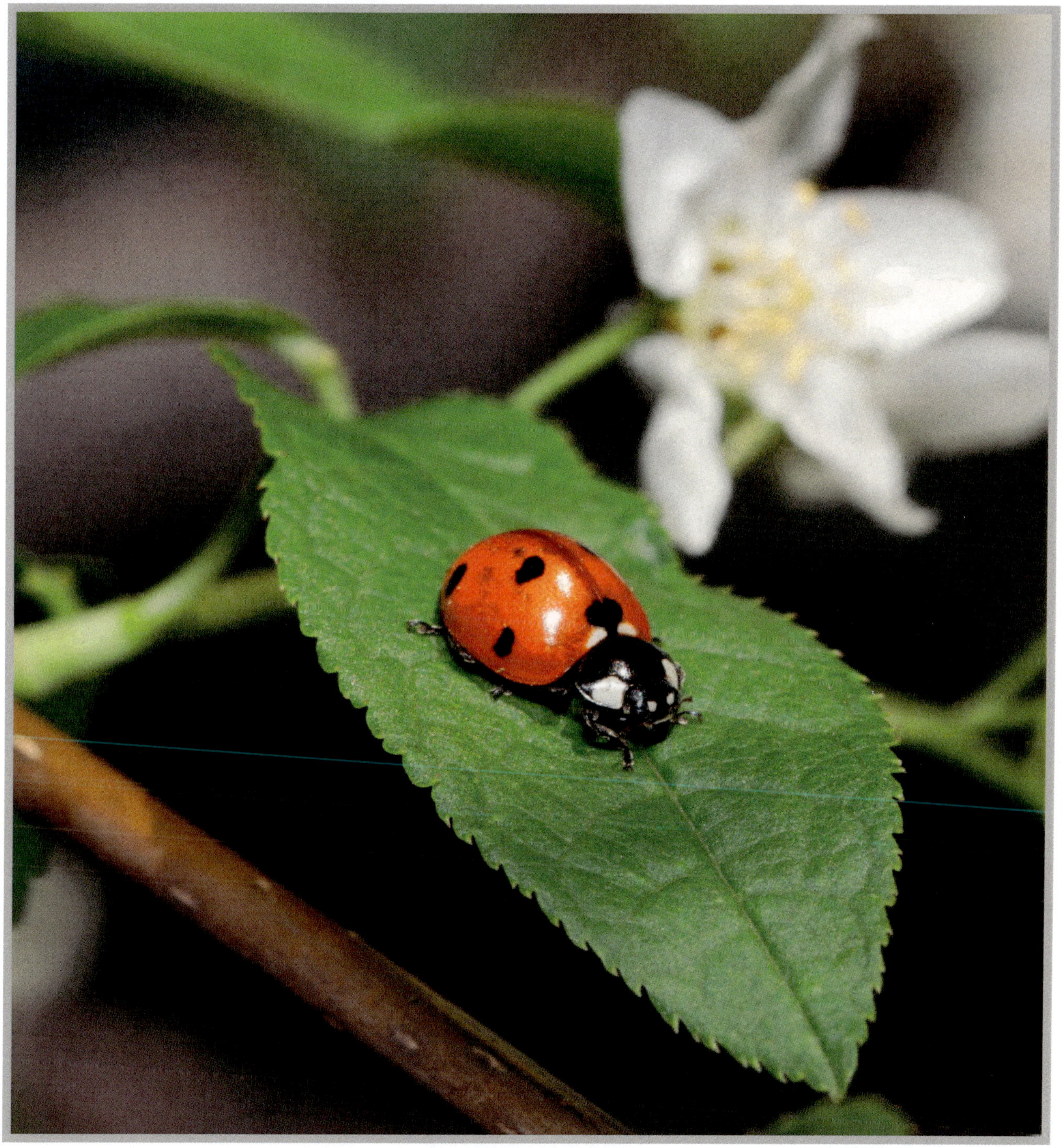

The Tyger

Tyger! Tyger! burning bright
In the forests of the night,
What immortal hand or eye
Could frame thy fearful symmetry?

William Blake

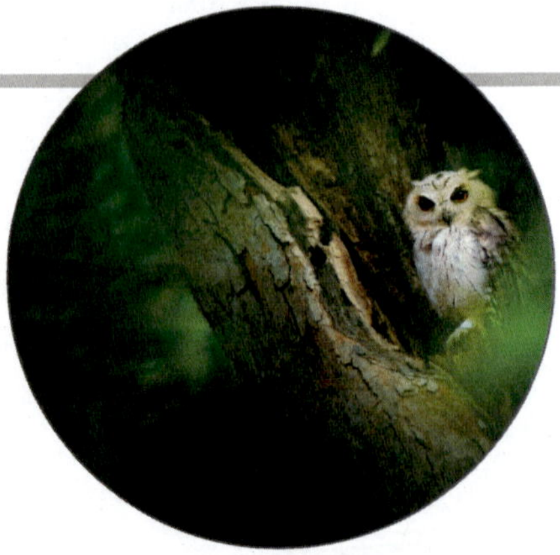

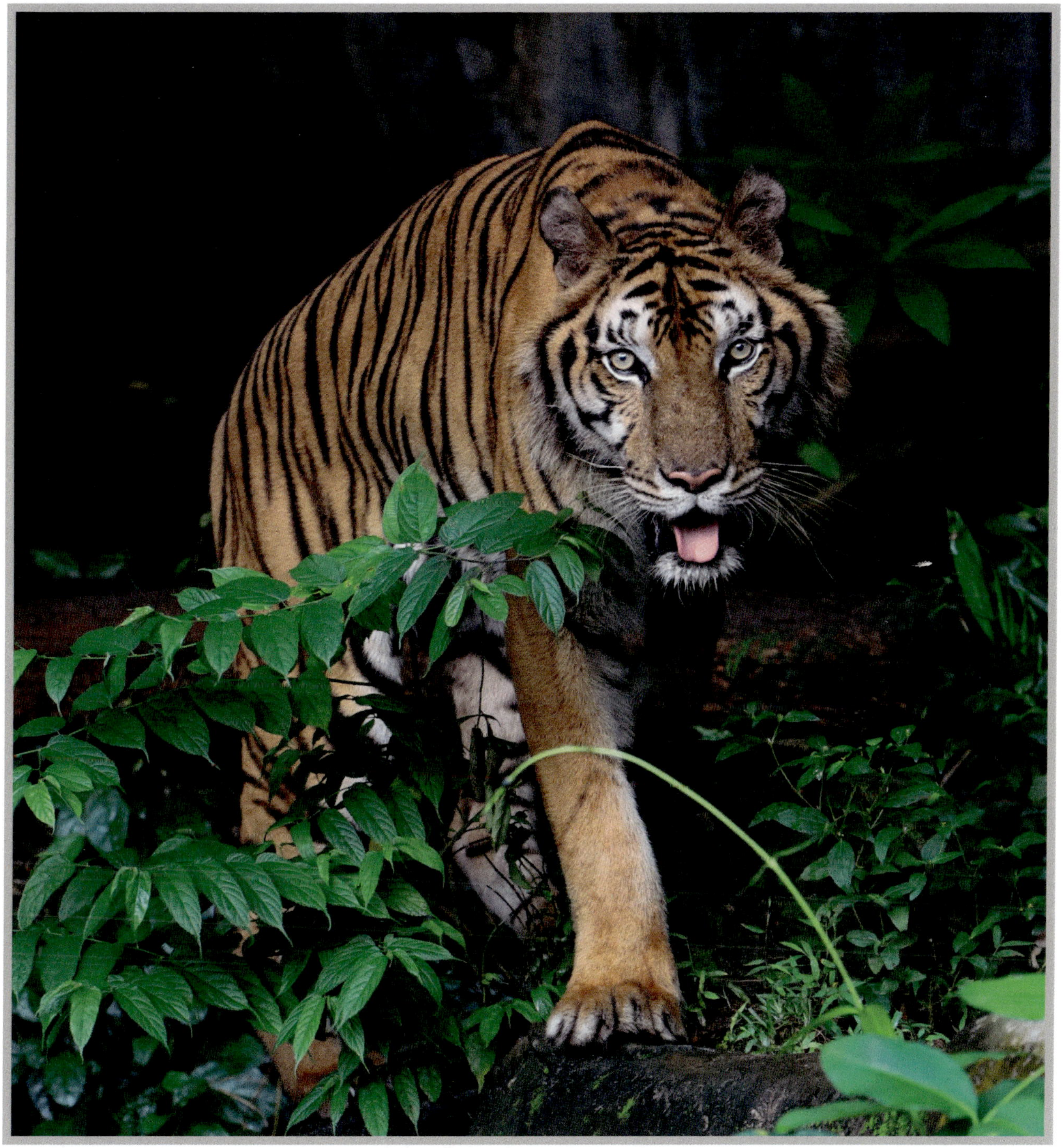

The Fieldmouse

Where the acorn tumbles down,
Where the ash tree sheds its berry,
With your fur so soft and brown,
With your eye so round and merry,
Scarcely moving the long grass,
Fieldmouse, I can see you pass.

Cecil Frances Alexander

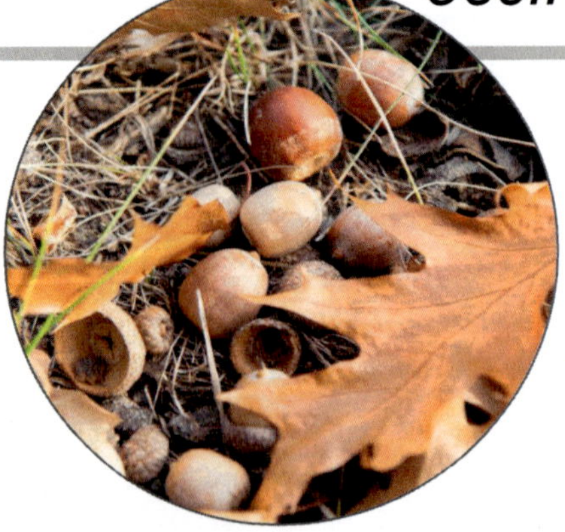

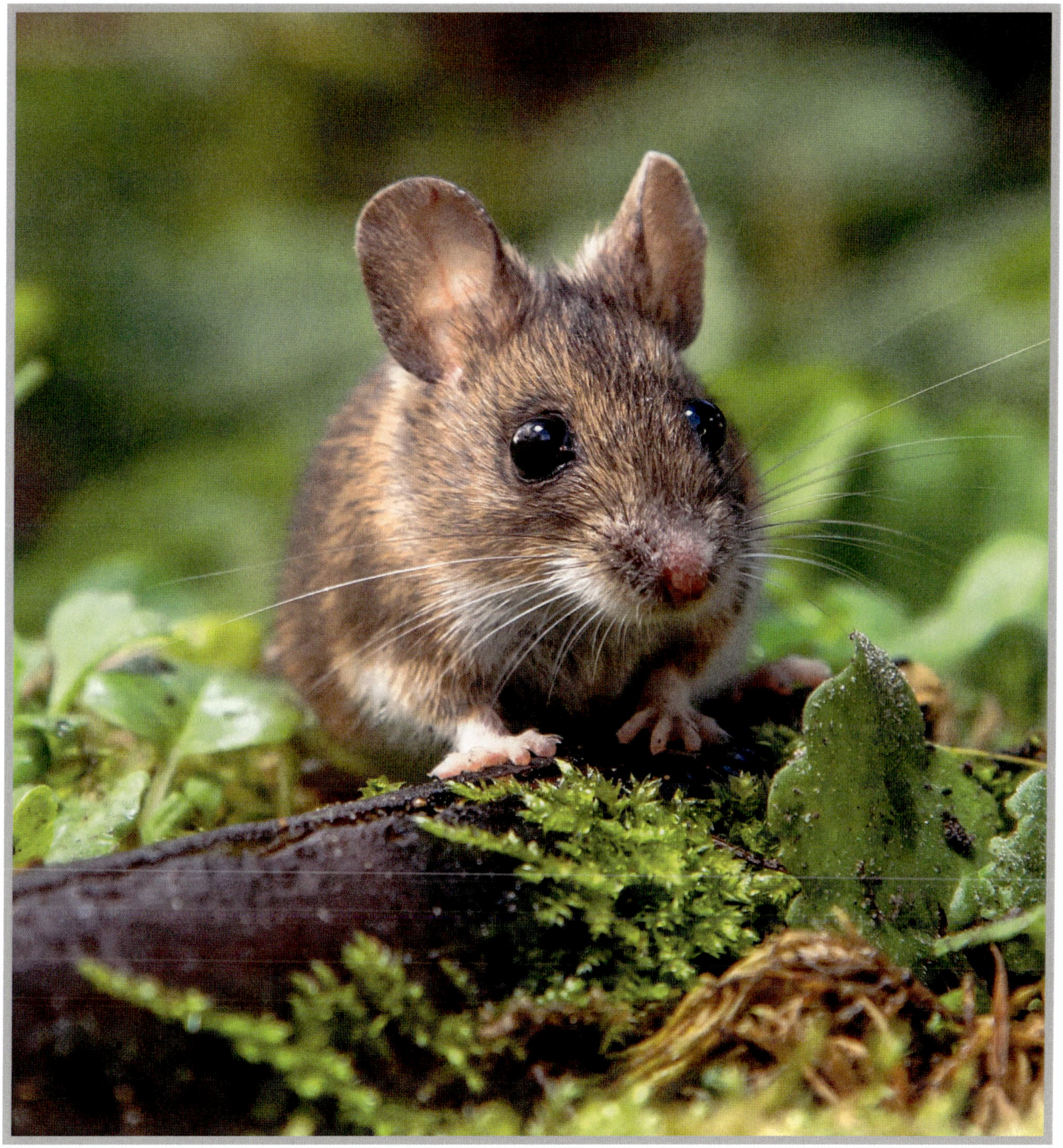

The Hairy Dog

My dog's so furry I've not seen
His face for years and years;
His eyes are buried out of sight,
I only guess his ears.
When people ask me for his breed,
I do not know or care;
He has the beauty of them all
Hidden beneath his hair.

Herbert Asquith

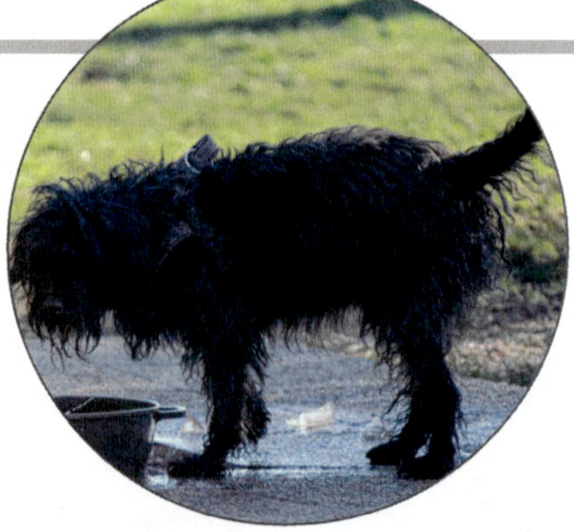

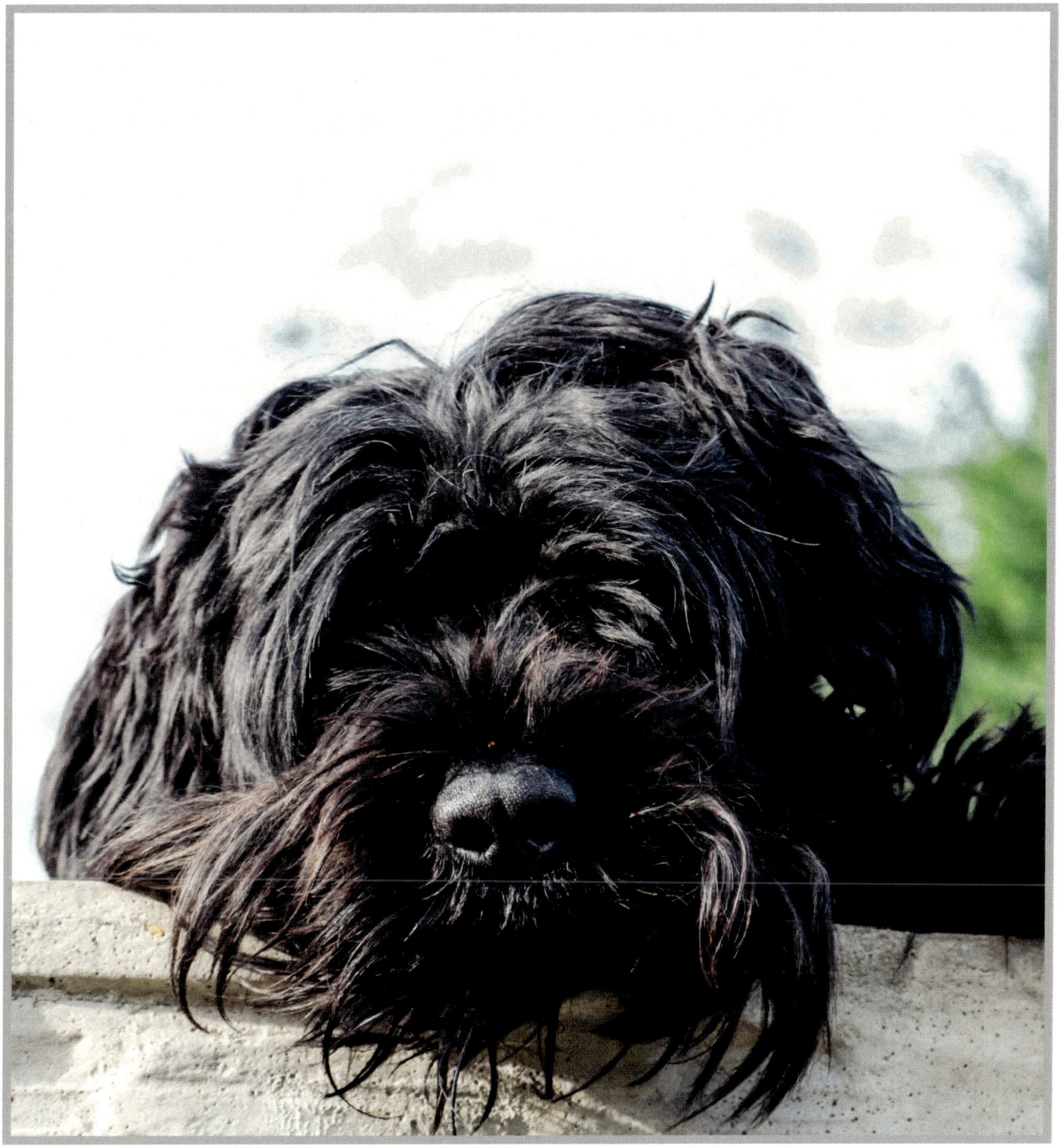

A Frisky Lamb

A frisky lamb
And a frisky child
Playing their pranks
In a cowslip meadow:
The sky all blue
And the air all mild
And the fields all sun
And the lanes half shadow.

Christina Rossetti

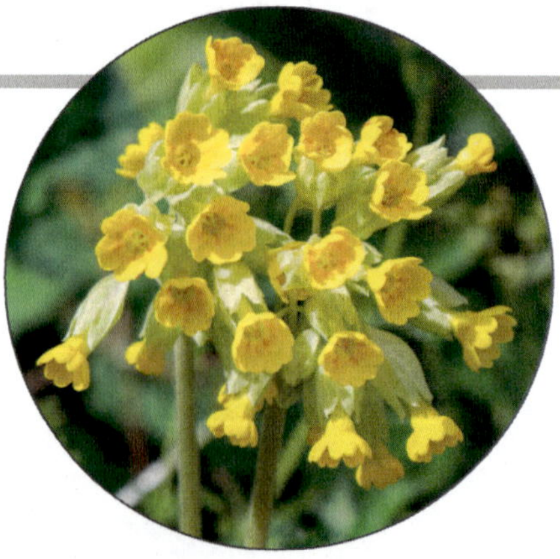

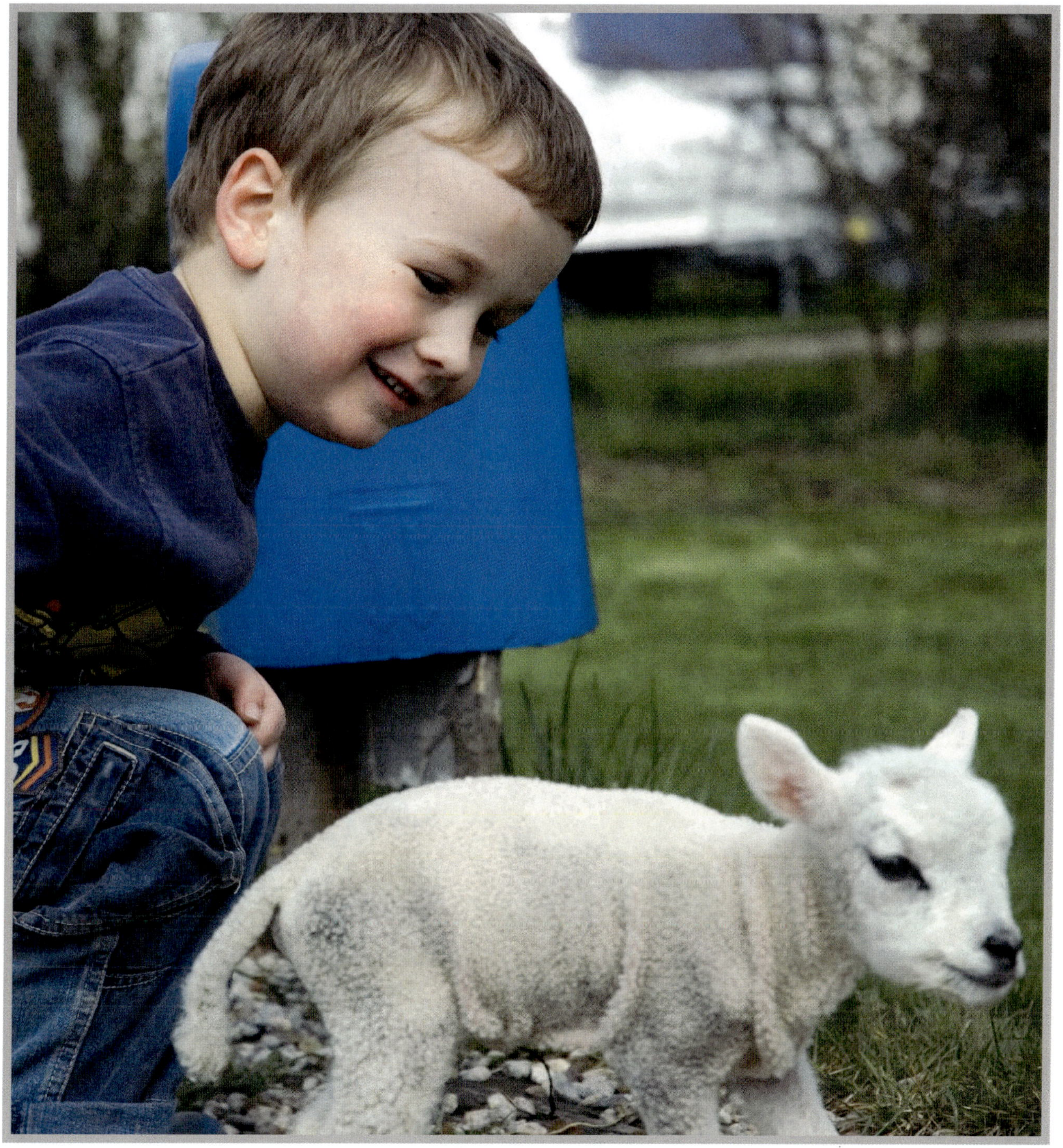

The Snail

To grass, or leaf, or fruit, or wall,
The snail sticks close, nor fears to fall,
As if he grew there, house and all
Together.

Where'er he dwells, he dwells alone,
Except himself has chattels none,
Well satisfied to be his own
Whole treasure.

William Cowper

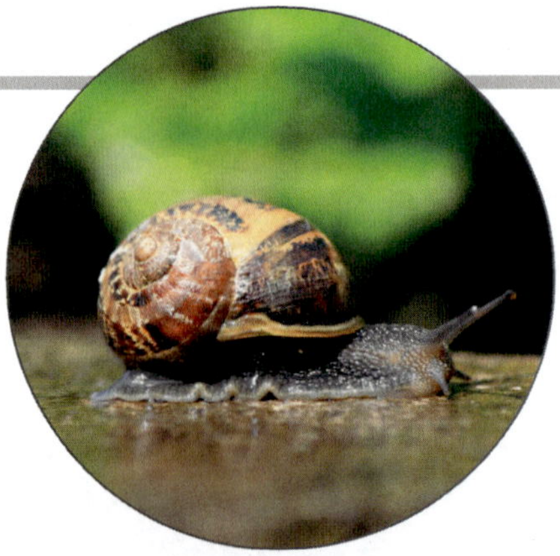

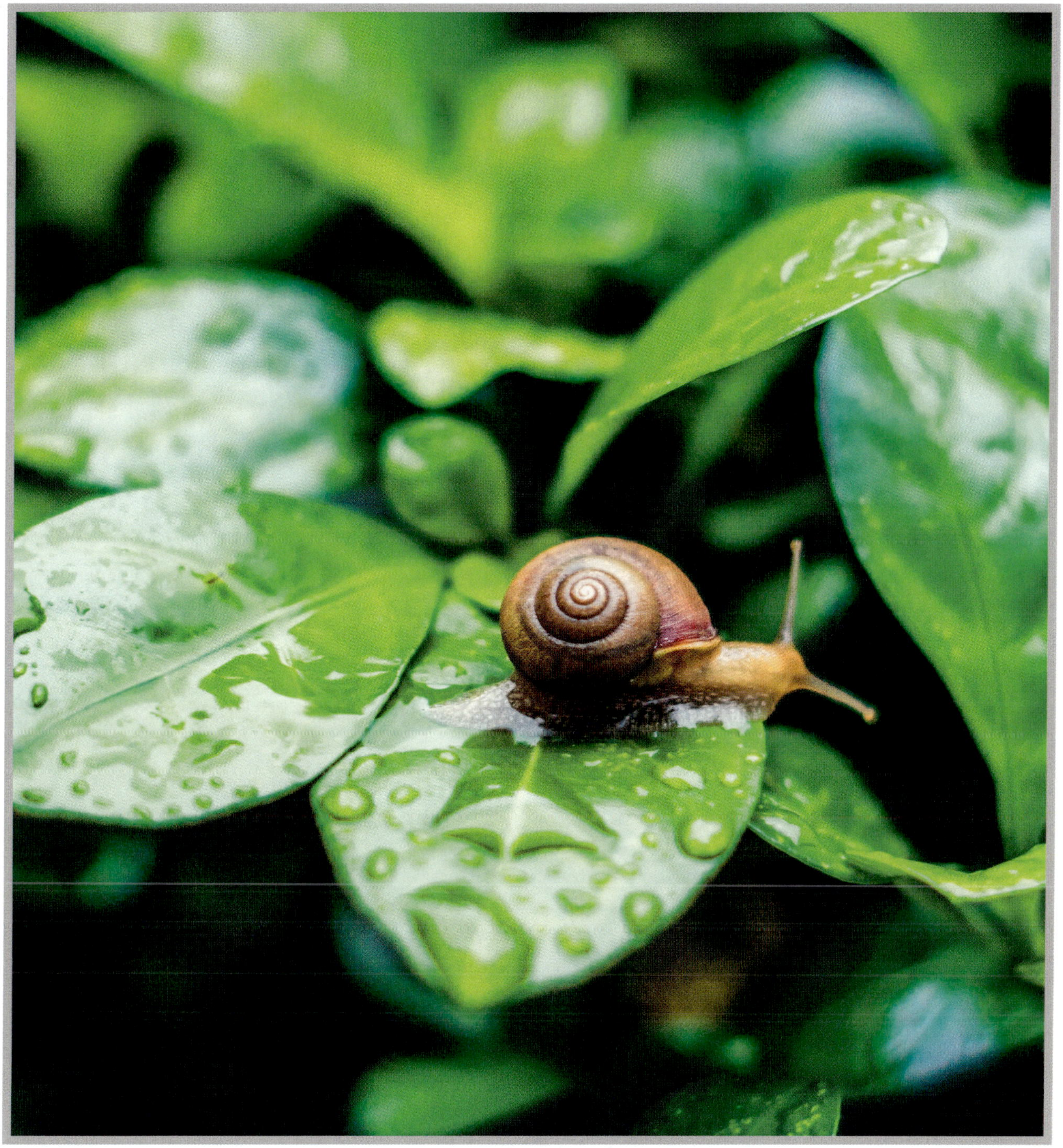

Hares at Play

The birds are gone to bed, the cows are still,
And sheep lie panting on each old mole hill;
And underneath the willow's grey-green bough
Like toil a-resting – lies the fallow plough.
The timid hares throw daylight's fears away
On the lane's road to dust and dance and play.

John Clare

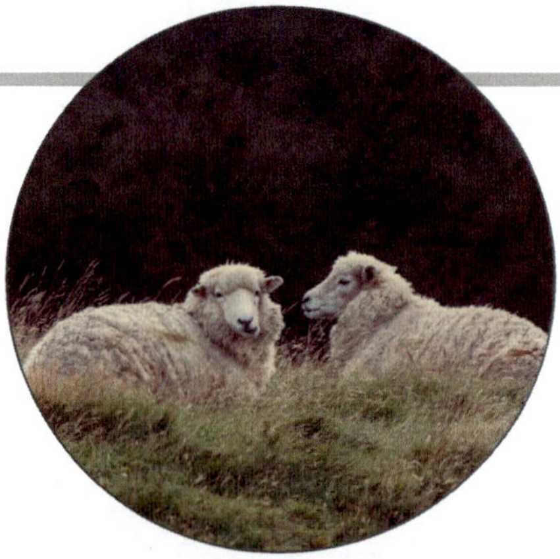

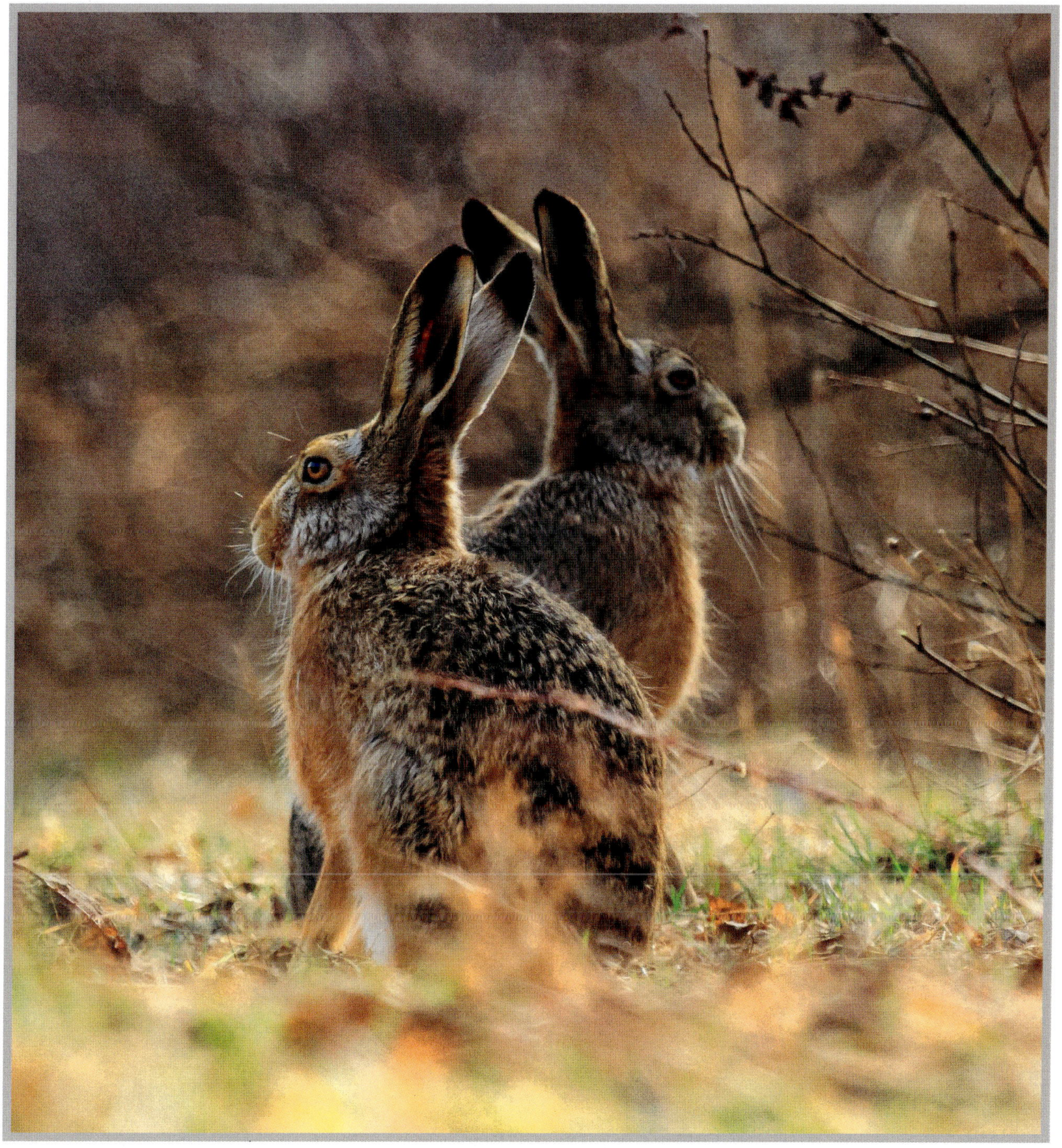

Milk for the Cat

When the tea is brought at five o'clock,
And all the neat curtains are drawn with care,
The little black cat with bright green eyes
Is suddenly purring there.

At first she pretends, having nothing to do,
She has come in merely to blink by the grate,
But, though tea may be late
Or the milk may be sour,
She is never late.

Harold Monro

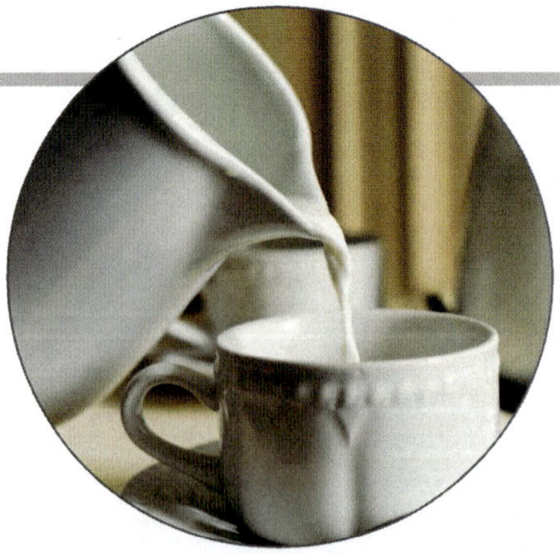

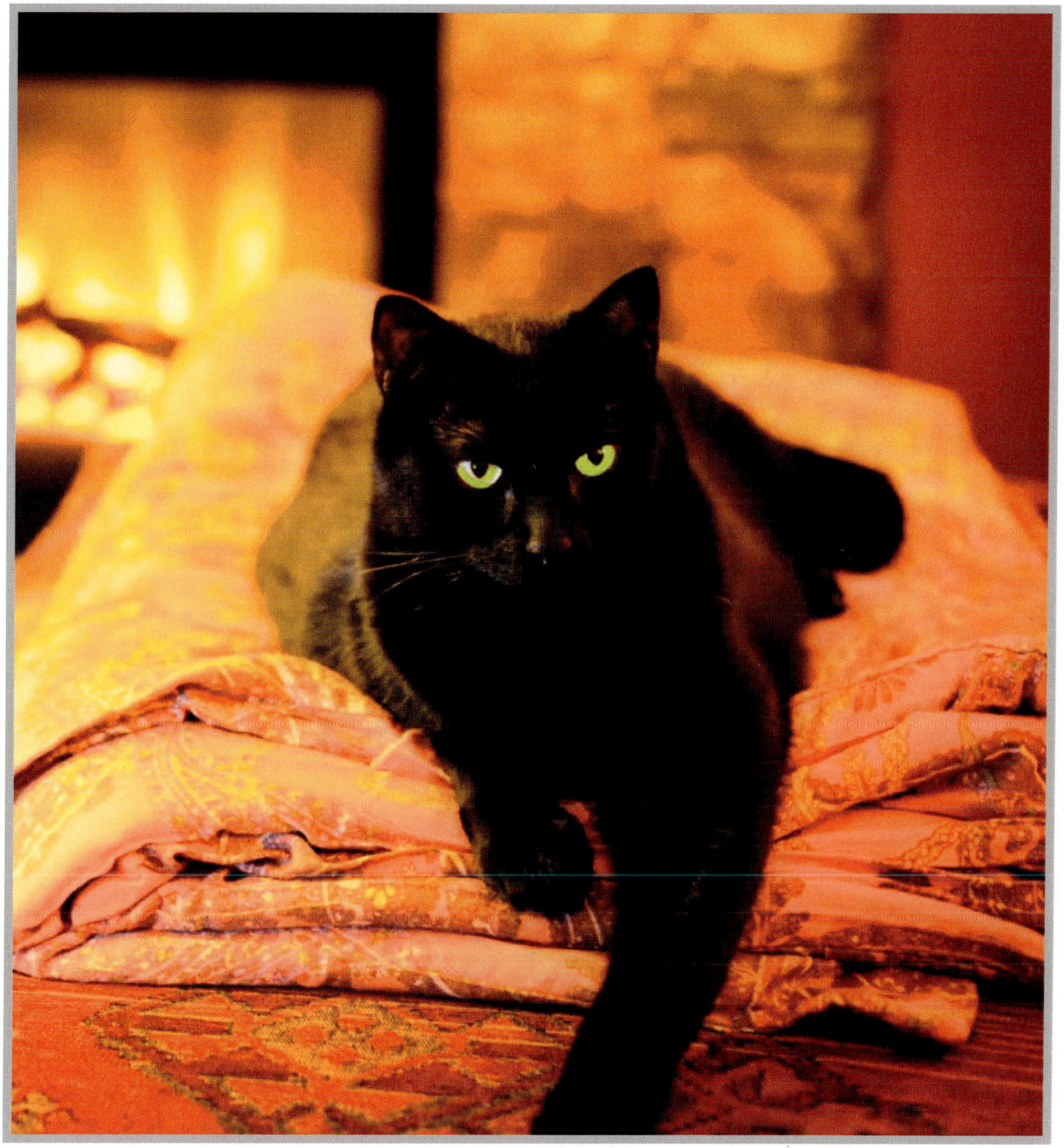

A Country Boy in Winter

I like to hear the old horse neigh
Just as I come in sight,
The oxen poke me with their horns
To get their hay at night.
Somehow the creatures seem like friends,
And like to see me come.
Some fellows talk about New York,
But I shall stay at home.

Sarah Orne Jewett

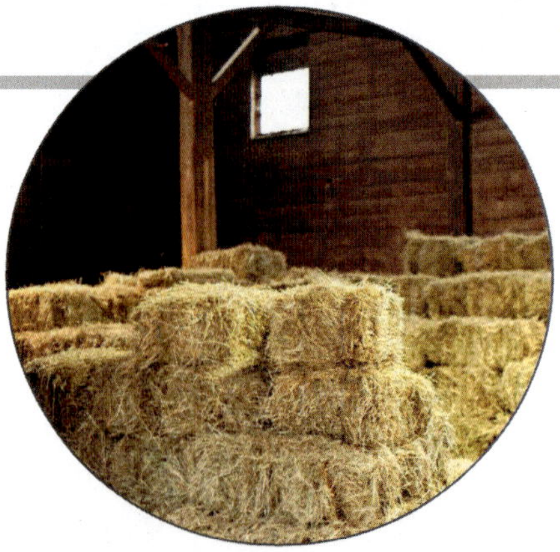

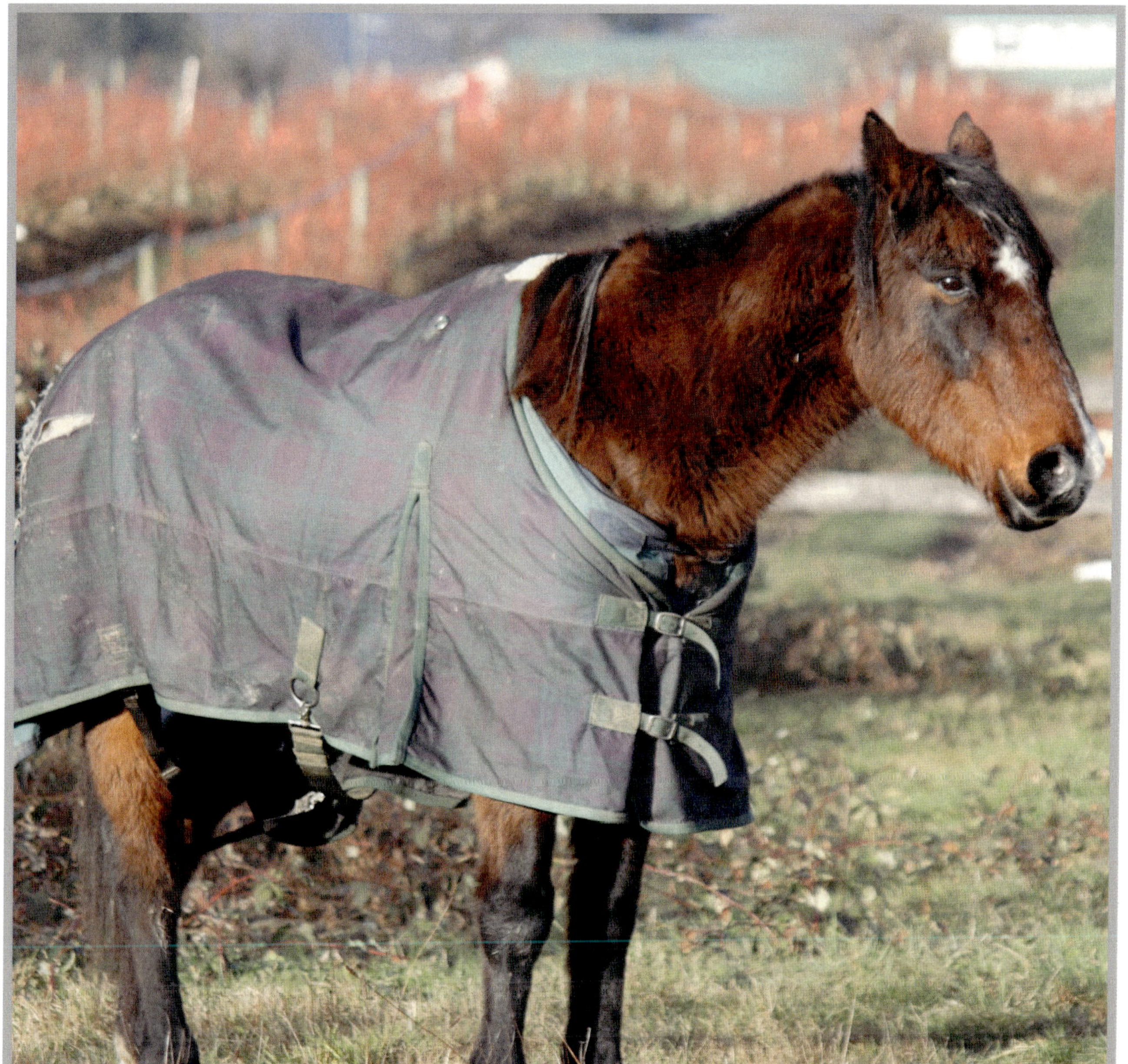

A Walk by the Water

Let us walk where reeds are growing,
By the alders in the mead;
Where the crystal streams are flowing,
In whose waves the fishes feed.

Do not dread us, timid fishes,
We have neither net nor hook;
Wanderers we, whose only wishes
Are to read in nature's book.

Charlotte Smith

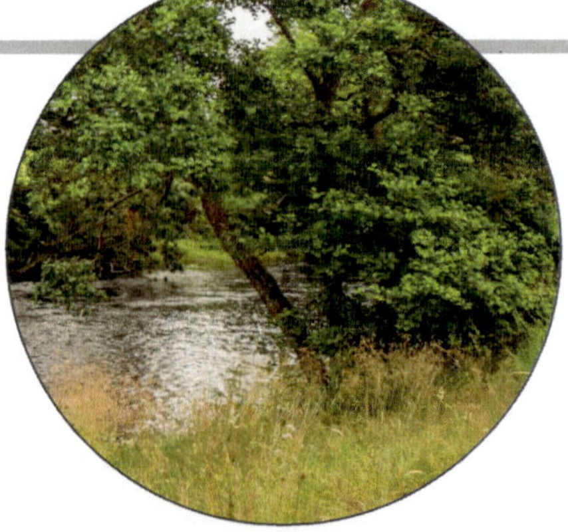

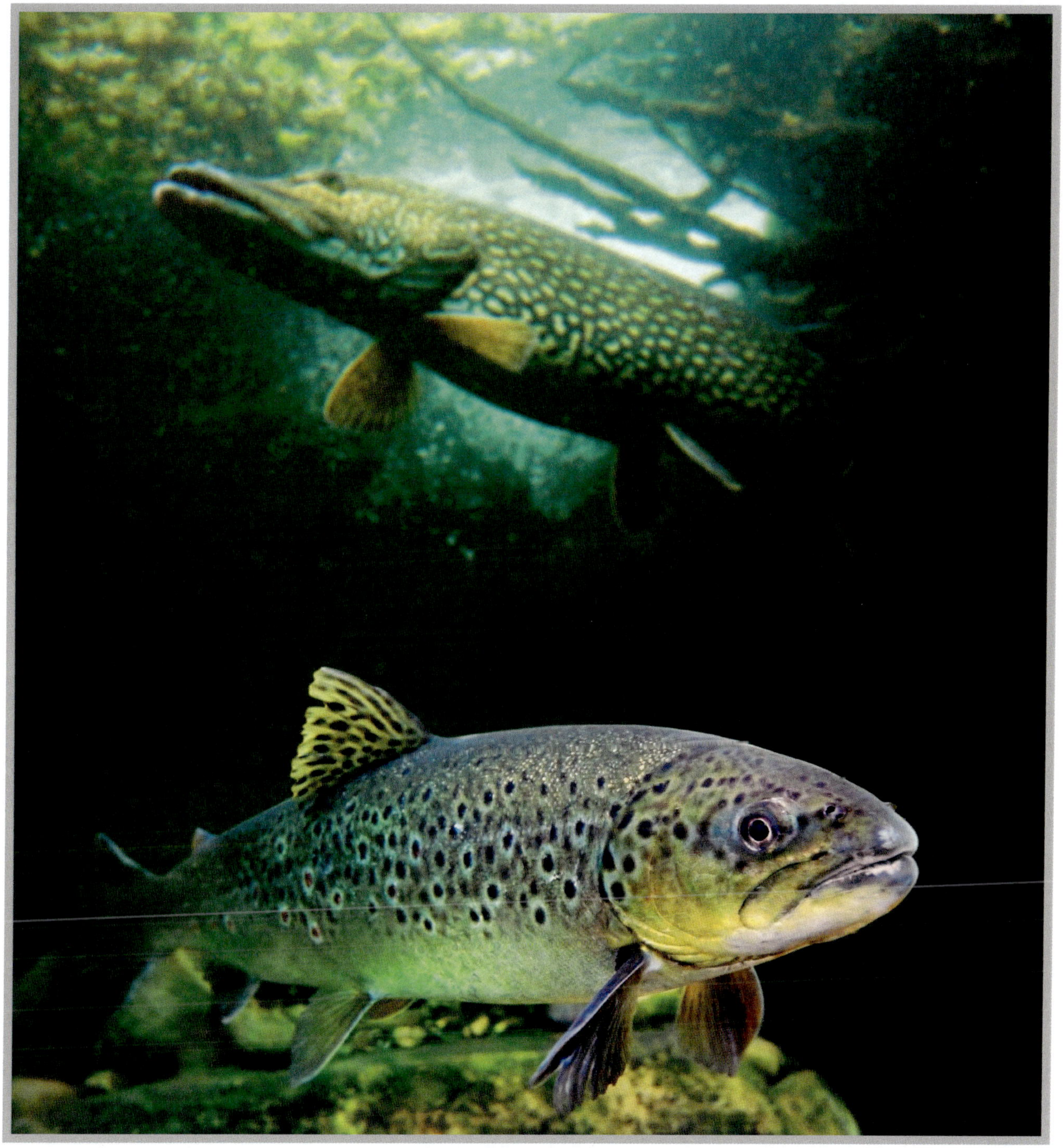

The Squirrel

Ay, there's the Squirrel perched aloft,
That active little rover;
See how he whisks his bushy tail,
Which shadows him all over;
Now rapid as a ray of light
He darts up yon tall beech;
He skips along from branch to branch;
And now the top can reach.

Sara Coleridge

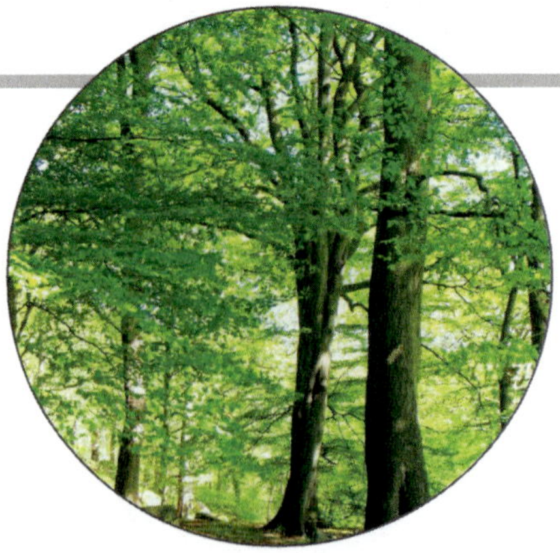

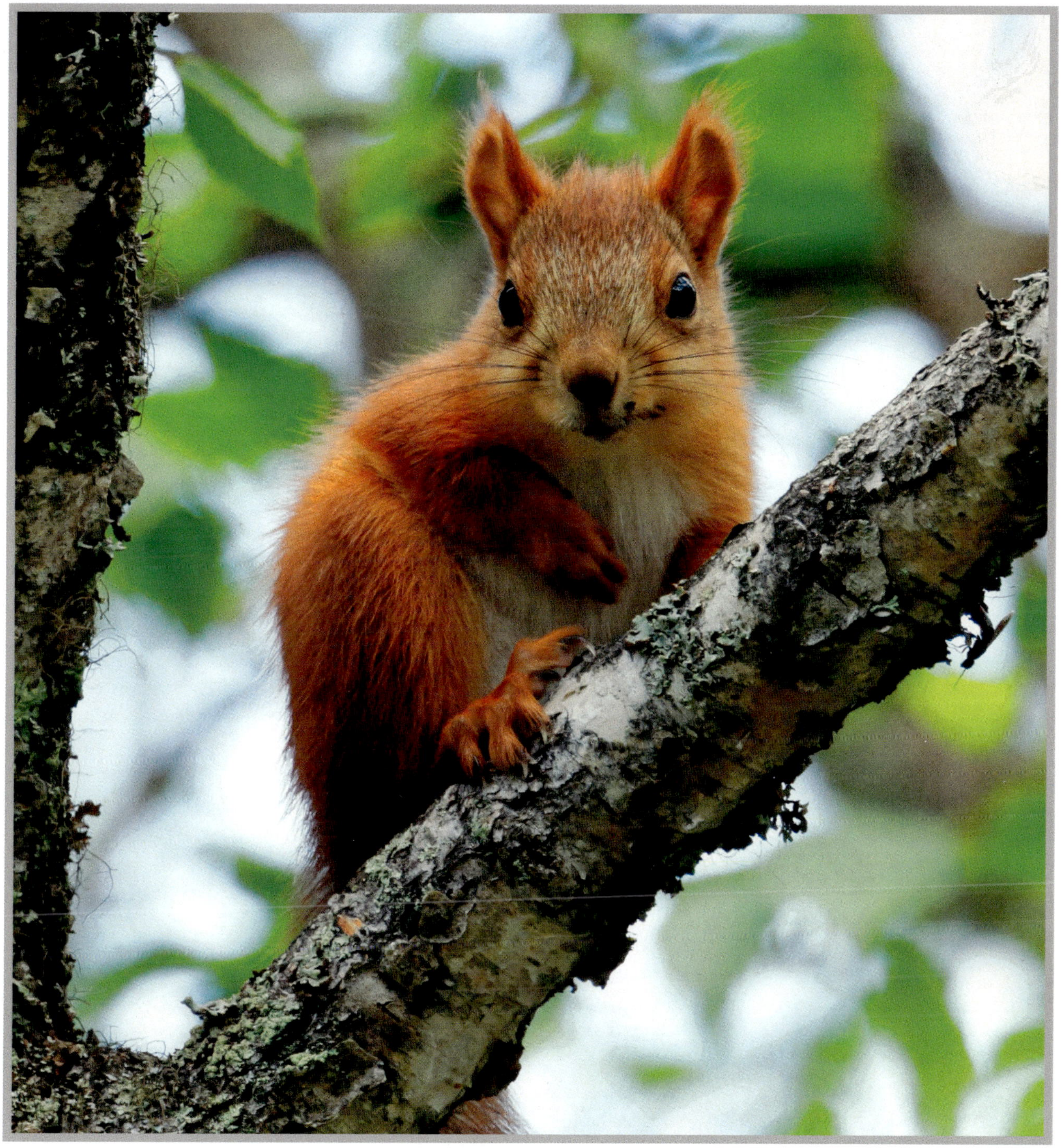

The Caterpillar

How soft a Caterpillar steps—
I find one on my Hand
From such a velvet world it comes
Such plushes at command
Its soundless travels just arrest
My slow terrestrial eye
Intent upon its own career
What use has it for me?

Emily Dickinson

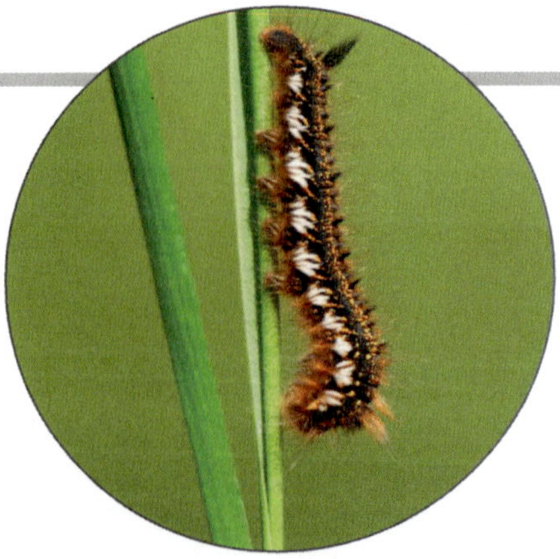

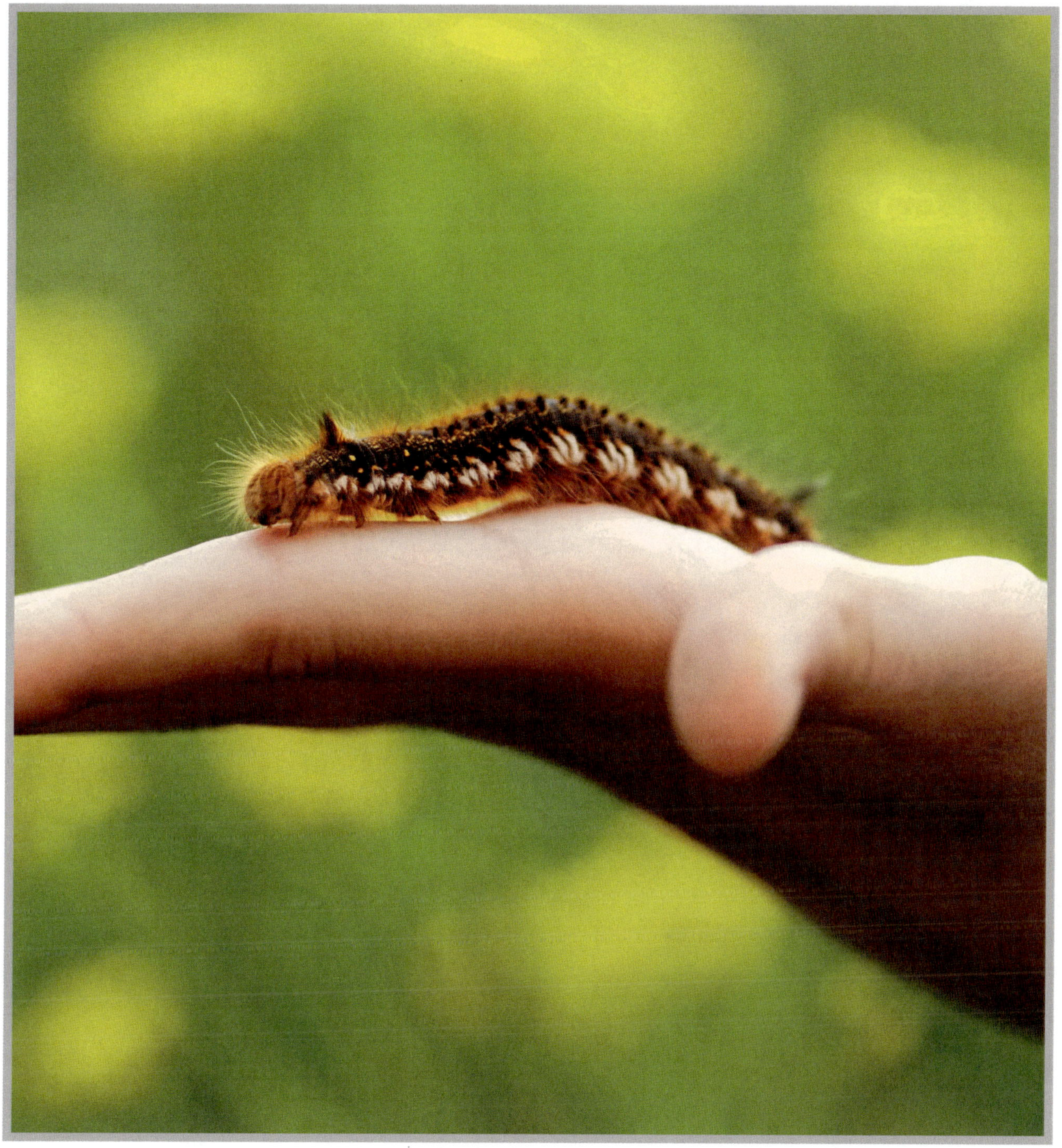

How doth the little busy bee

How doth the little busy bee
Improve each shining hour,
And gather honey all the day
From every opening flower!

How skilfully she builds her cell!
How neat she spreads the wax!
And labours hard to store it well
With the sweet food she makes.

Isaac Watts

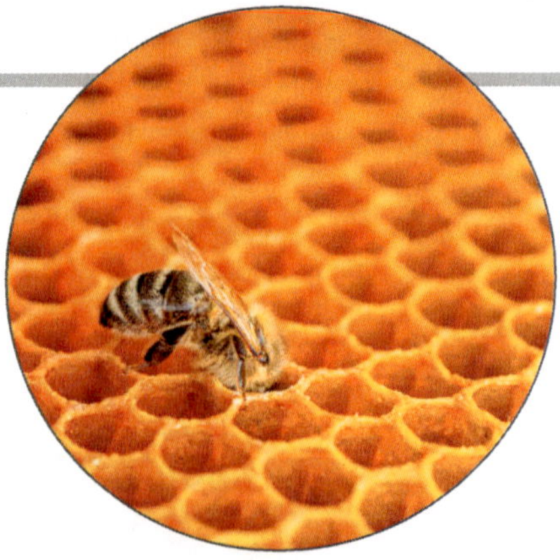

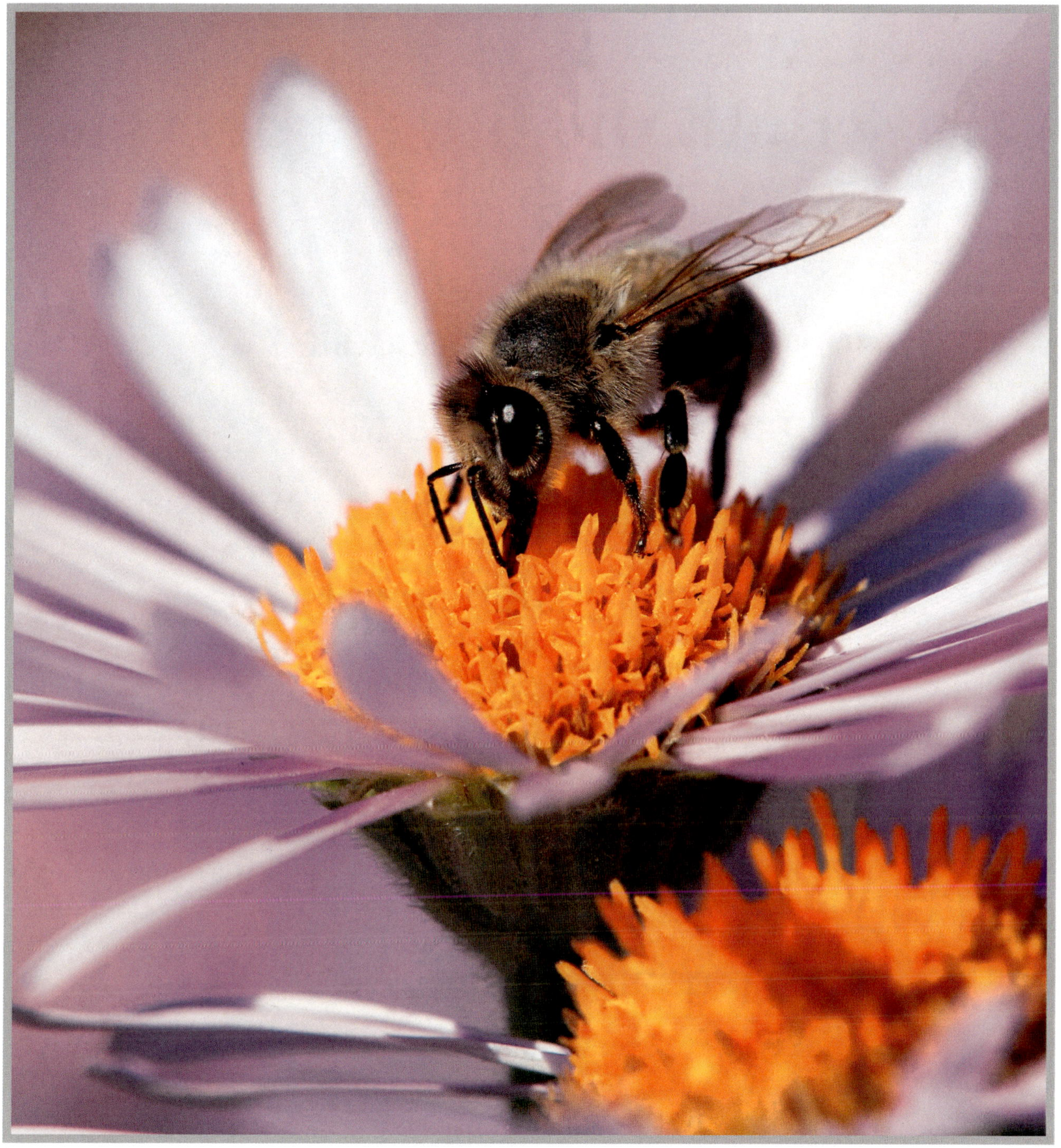

How doth the little crocodile

(A parody)

How doth the little crocodile
Improve his shining tail,
And pour the waters of the Nile
On every golden scale!

How cheerfully he seems to grin,
How neatly spreads his claws,
And welcomes little fishes in,
With gently smiling jaws!

Lewis Carroll

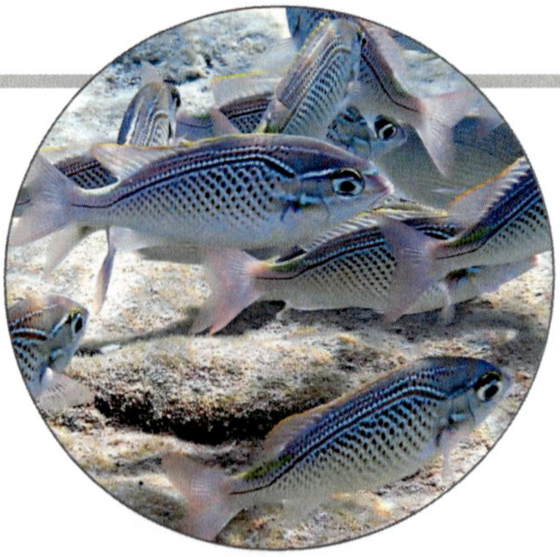

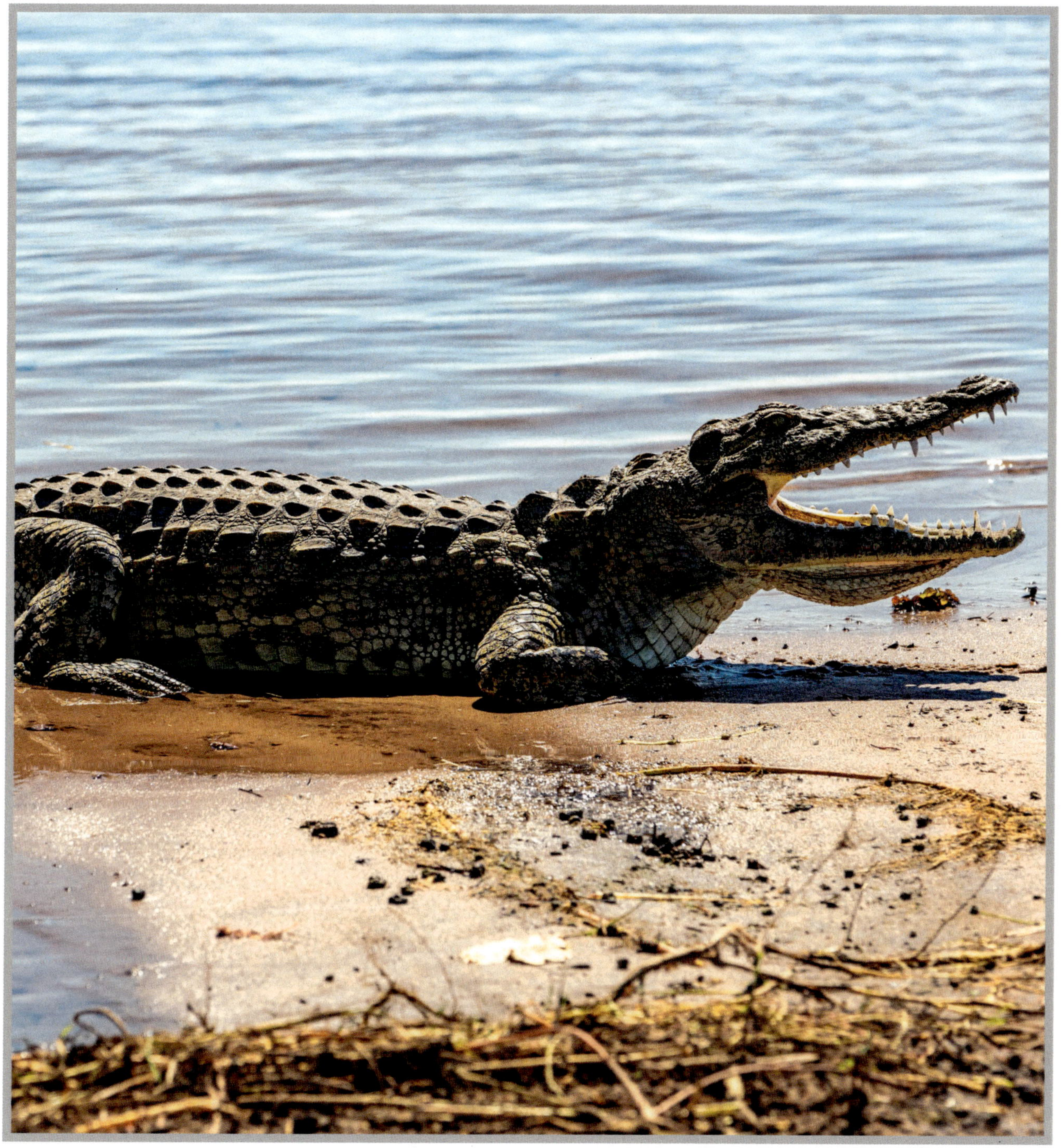

The Lizard

Jewelled Lizard, you and I
On the heathery hill-top lie,
While the westering sun inclines
Past the clump of red-stemmed pines;
O’er the little space of sun
Creep their shadows, one by one.

A. C. Benson

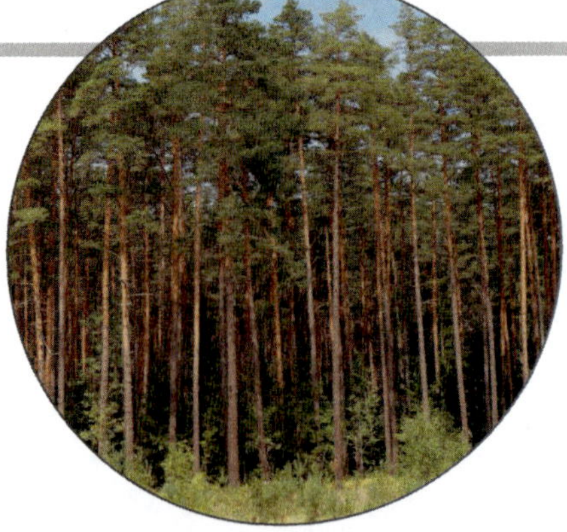

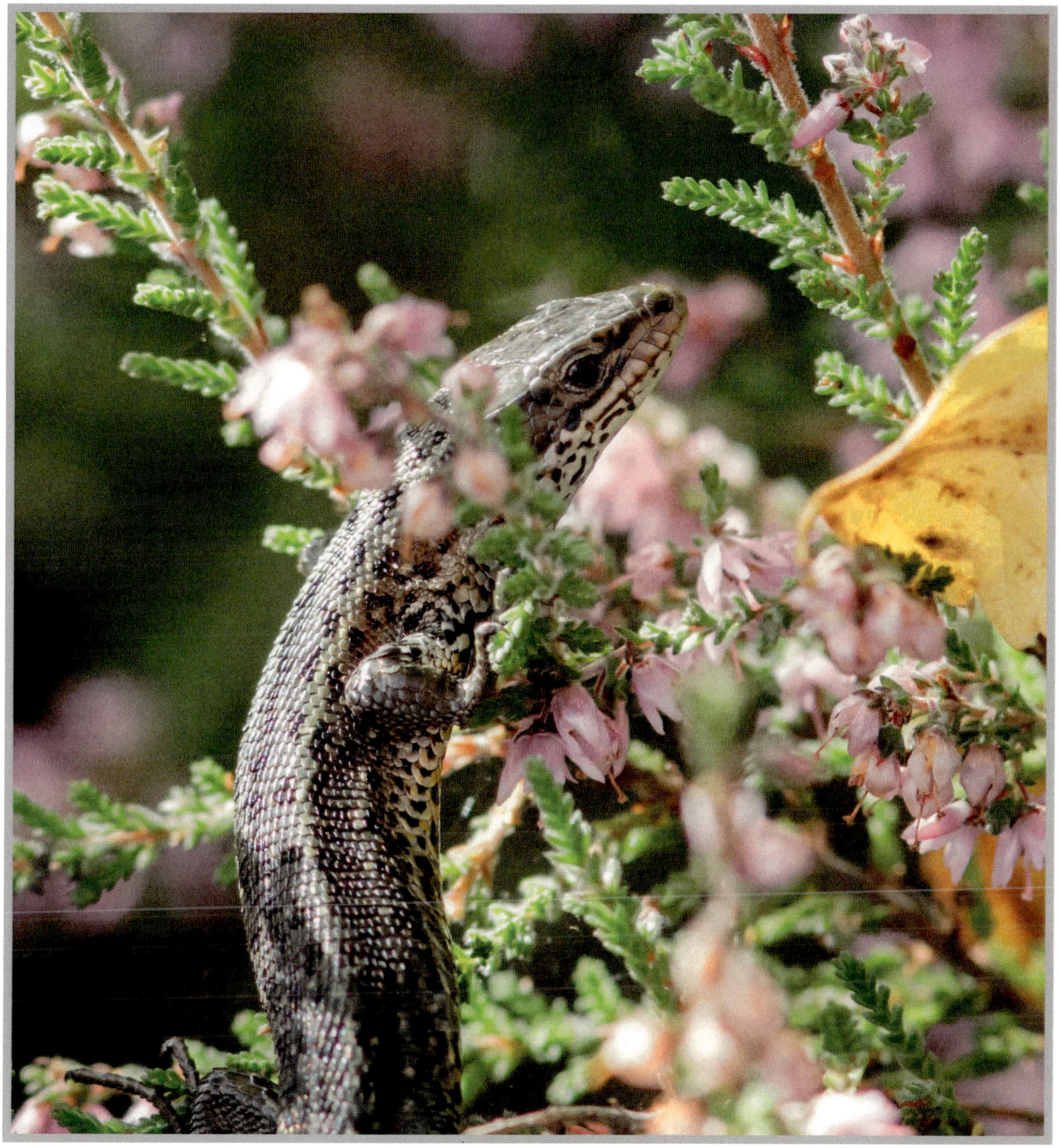

Lullaby for Titania
(A Midsummer Night's Dream)

Ye spotted snakes with double tongue,
Thorny hedgehogs, be not seen;
Newts and blindworms, do no wrong,
Come not near our fairy Queen.
Philomele, with melody
Sing in our sweet lullaby;
Lulla, lulla, lullaby,
Lulla, lulla, lullaby.

William Shakespeare

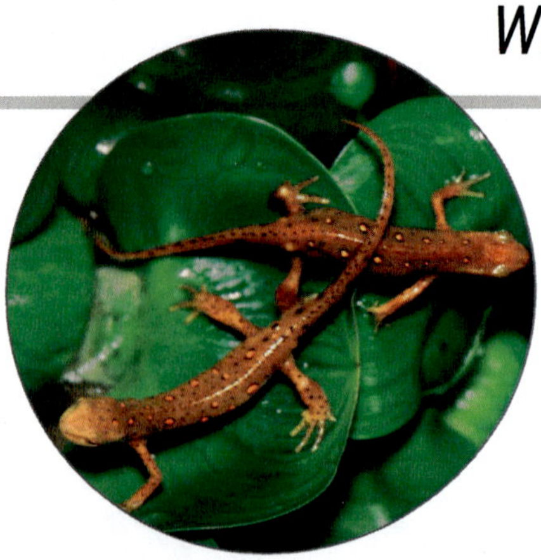

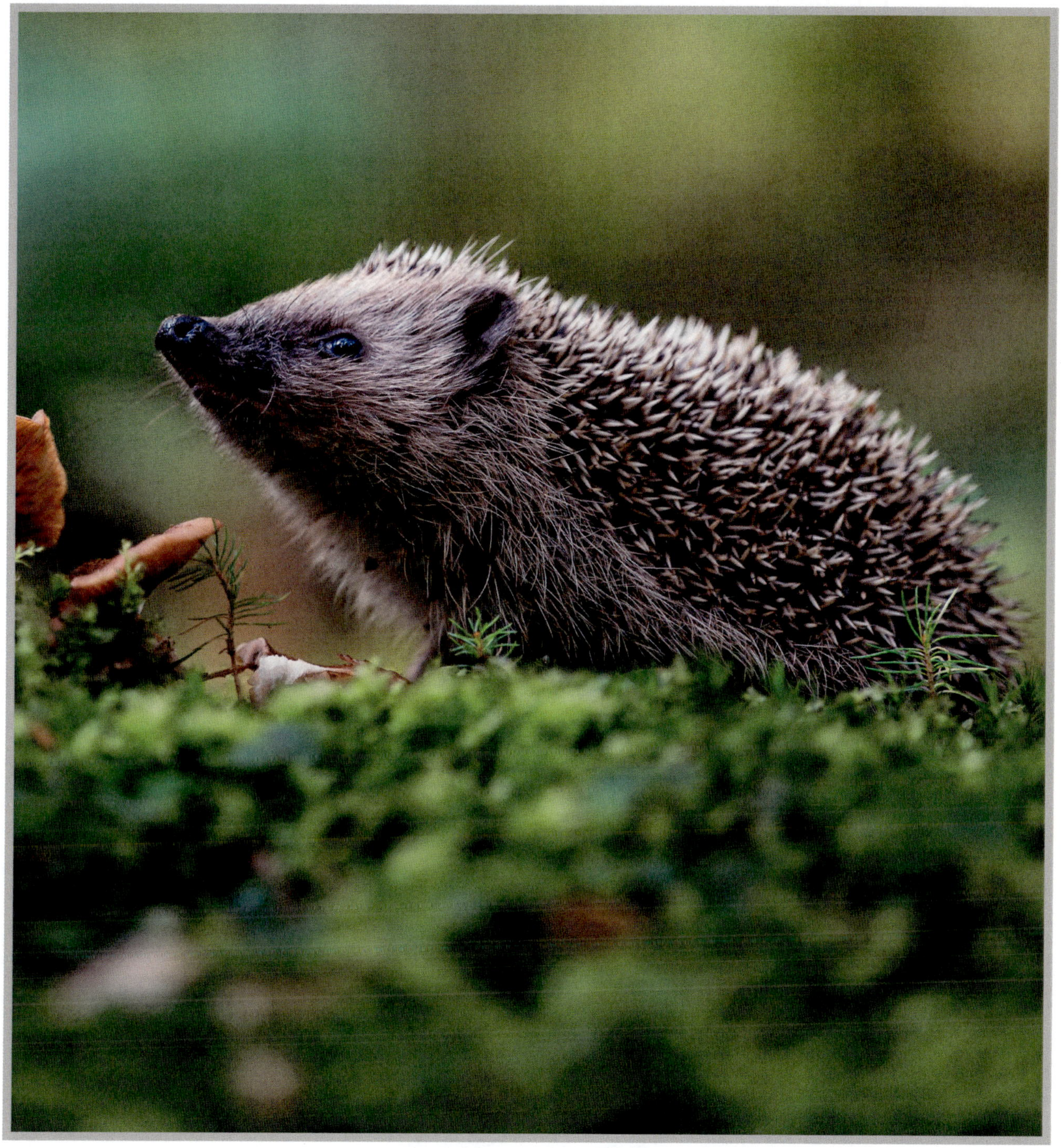

The Example

Here's an example from
A Butterfly—That on a rough, hard rock
Happy can lie;
Friendless and all alone
On this unsweetened stone.

Now let my bed be hard—No care take I;
I'll make my joy like this
Small Butterfly;
Whose happy heart has power
To make a stone a flower.

W. H. Davies

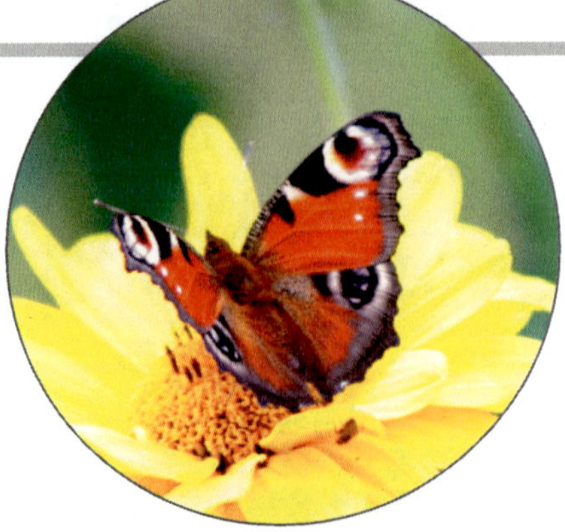

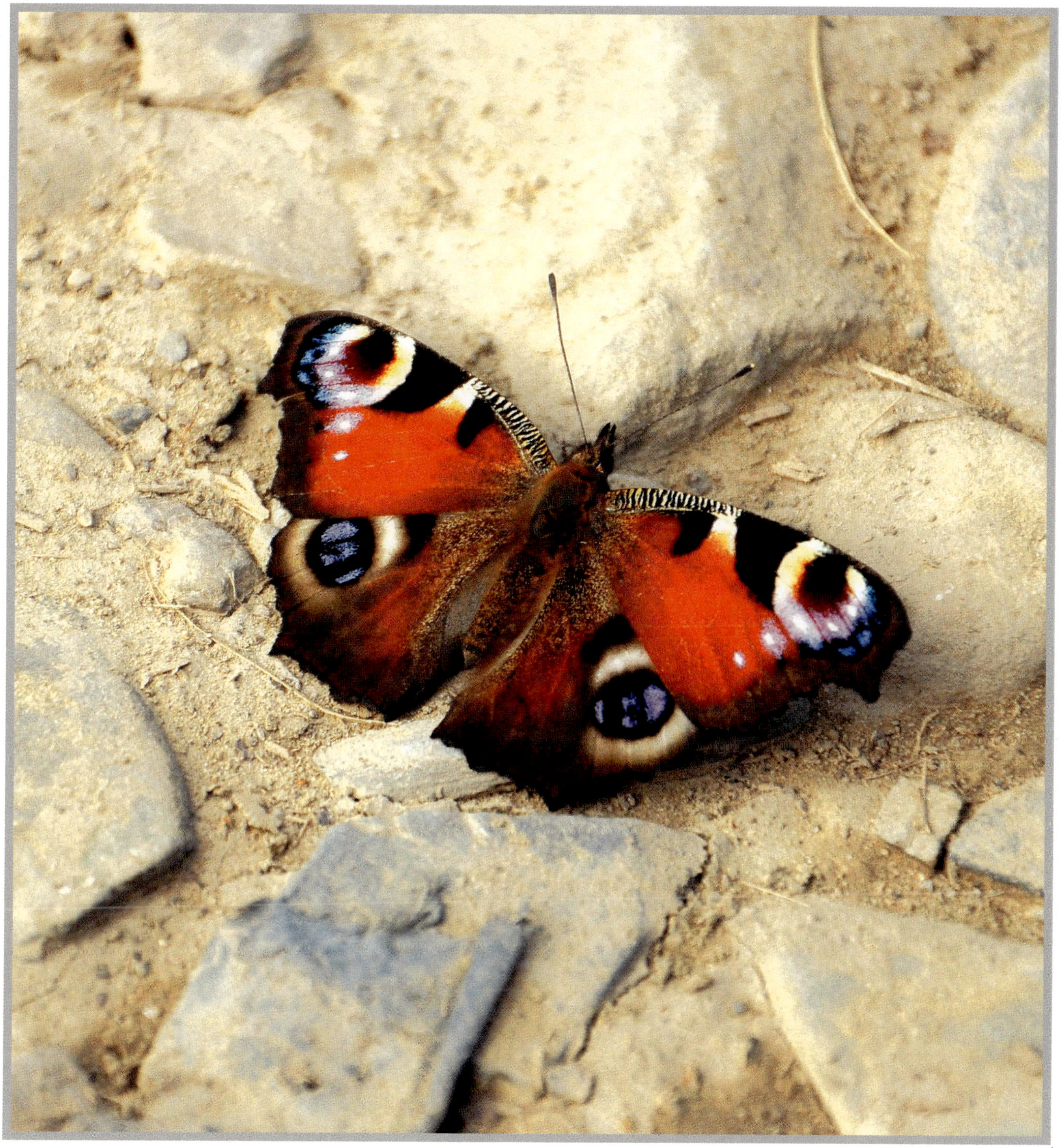

The Deer

Under the pines and the hemlocks
The thick, white cloud mists creep,
And drip all down the needles brown
Where the dun deer lies asleep.
Follow, follow, by hill and hollow,
The doe to her spotted fawn;
'Tis dark o' the moon,
But day comes soon
For I sniff the breath of the dawn.

Mary Austin

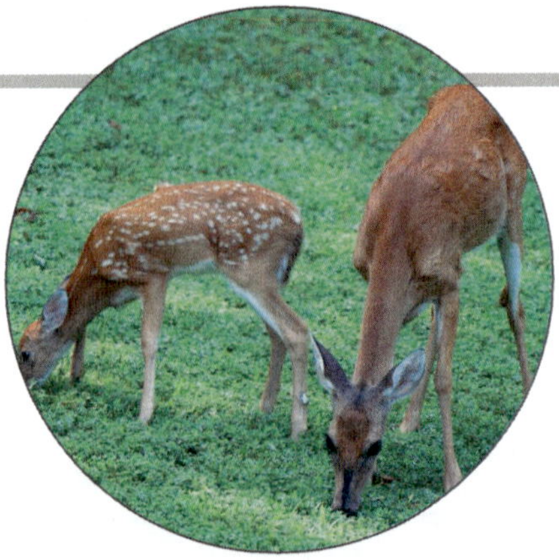

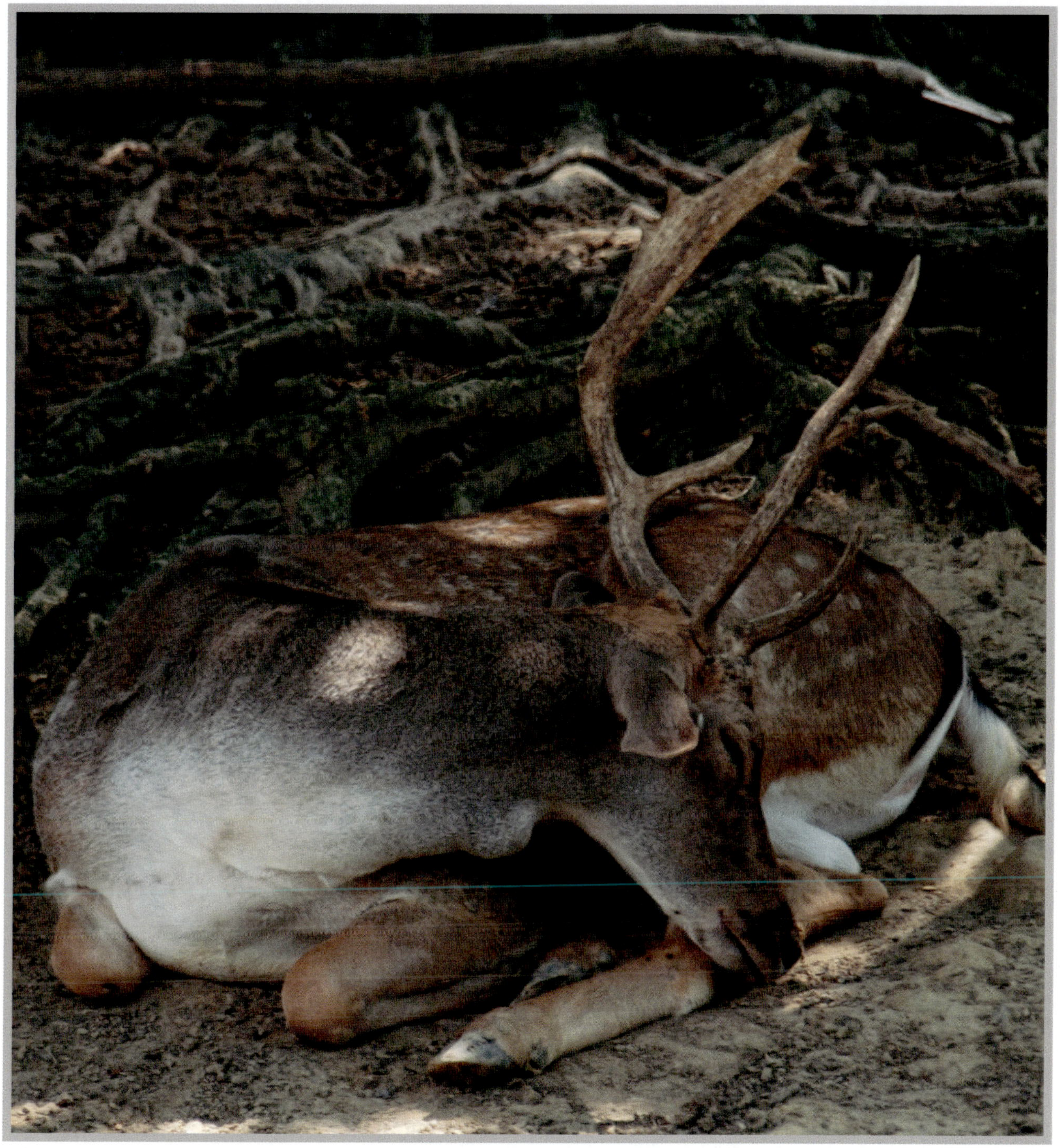

Our Cow

Down by the sliprails stands our cow
　Chewing, chewing, chewing,
She does not care what folks out there
　In the great, big world are doing.
She sees the small cloud-shadows pass
　And green grass shining under.
If she does think, what does she think
　About it all, I wonder?

C. J. Dennis

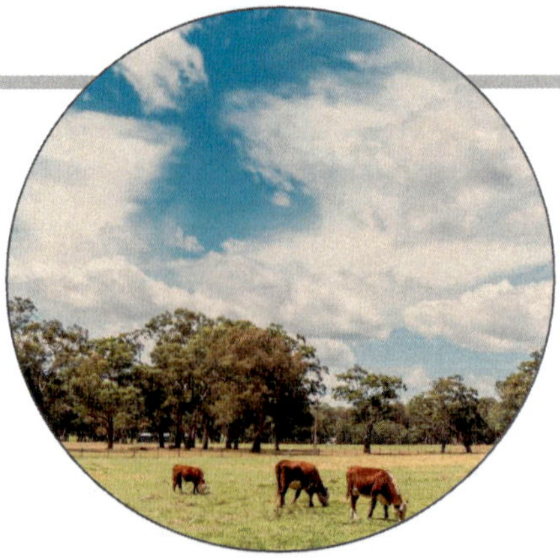

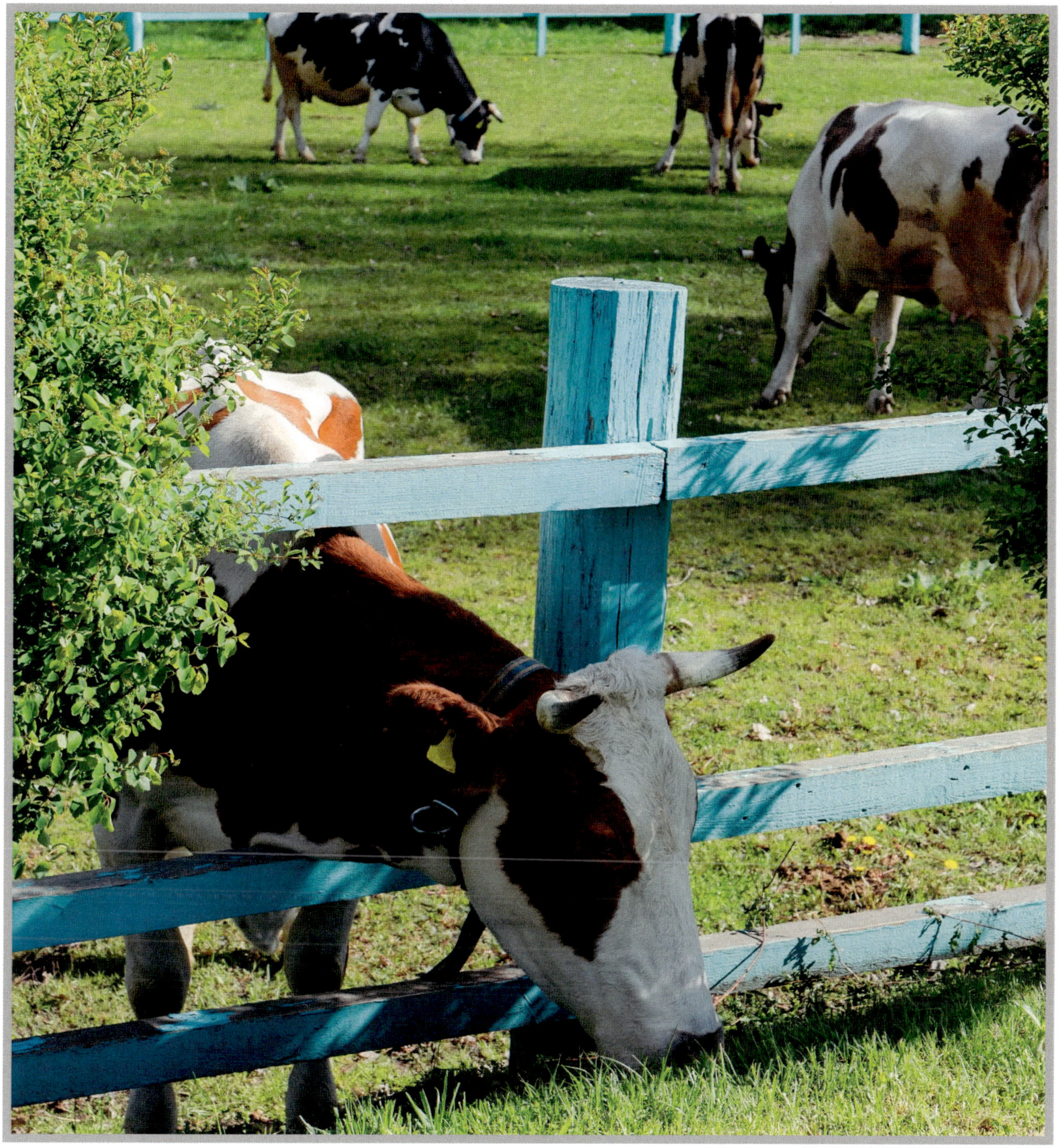

Thank you for reading!
You might also enjoy:

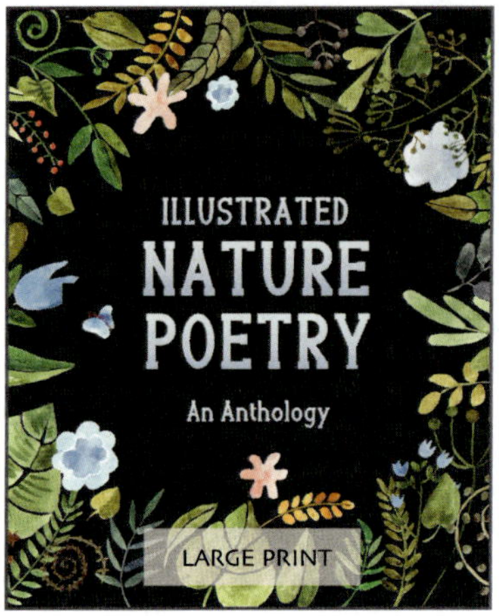

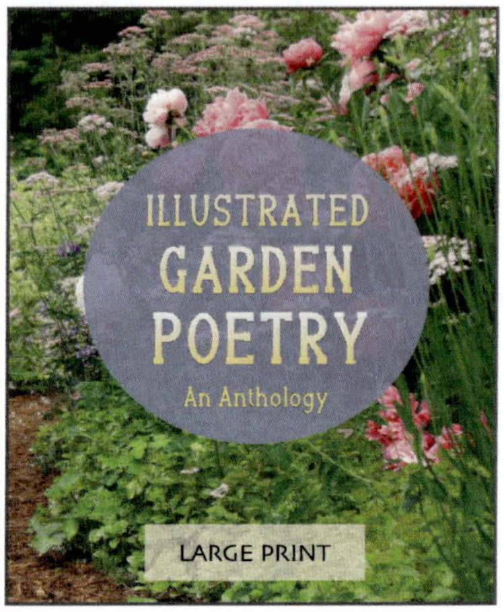

Huge thanks to Alison Egan (professional advice)
and Emma Laybourn, Jennifer J. Barwick (editing).

All these poems are in the Public Domain. Photos from Deposit Photos:
Armastus, catstyecam, davem1972, Sergey Tikhomirov, OndrejProsicky, pumppump, stetsik, CreativeNature, Columbo, JanRozehnal, tommeaker26, mamopictures, naffarts, galitskaya, Kamchatka, TSpider, nito103, Tepic, elenathewise, modfos, SnapTPhotography, vladvitek, Philopenshaw, Giedriius, sstandbridge, Dimedrol68, christening, prudek, gorsh13, Panthermediaseller, Hans_Chr, shaftinaction, DesignPics, RudolfPrchlik, PantherMediaSeller, Cirera, gsagi, ldambies, moisseyev, anmbph

Made in the USA
Coppell, TX
05 November 2026

11302978R00026